POLYCYSTIC
LIVER DISEASE

Information for Patients

By David Drum

Burning Books Press
Wellness Edition

First print edition ISBN # 978-0-9911857-6-4
Cover design by Karrie Ross, Be It Now and Arthur Kegerris.
http://polycysticliverdisease.weebly.com/

Burning Books Press
Wellness Edition

For Amy

TABLE OF CONTENTS

AUTHOR'S PREFACE

When my daughter was diagnosed with polycystic liver disease, I knew very little about it. To my knowledge, neither polycystic liver disease nor its frequent companion, polycystic kidney disease, had occurred in our family before. When my daughter began to experience the very common symptom of pain from an enlarged liver, she asked me to help her. As a medical journalist and the author of several health books, I began to learn about what was to me an unfamiliar and somewhat rare disease.

It was not easy to find much basic information for the patient with polycystic liver disease. There was a little information on the internet. Medical journals contained the most reliable data, but this information was scattered over many different publications and written for an audience of sophisticated medical professionals.

Eventually, my daughter was able to make an informed choice on a medical treatment for her pain. After a battle with her health insurance company, and a trip to the Mayo Clinic for a second opinion, happily, the surgery she chose turned out well. For the benefit of others in my daughter's situation, I decided to condense the information I found into this short book.

We live in an age when many people wish to be active partners in their medical treatment. However, being diagnosed with a chronic disease can be frightening and unsettling. Panic can set in when the patient faces medical treatment choices that they don't fully understand. To make good decisions in our complex medical system, we need good information. And unfortunately, medical doctors do not always have the time to fully answer complex questions or to completely explain everything a particular patient might wish to know.

Polycystic Liver Disease: Information for Patients contains background and treatment information for the person with polycystic liver disease. The book includes a simple explanation of the disease, the role of the liver in the body, symptoms and complications which may occur, and identified risk factors. A good deal of nutritional information is included. For fine-tuning the dietary information presented here, I am grateful for the assistance of registered dietitians Nickie Francisco-Ziller, RD, and Sara Di Cecco, MS, RD, of the Mayo Clinic, in Rochester, Minnesota, one of the institutions leading the way in finding new treatments for this puzzling disease.

Polycystic Liver Disease: Information for Patients contains helpful information on exercise, lifestyle issues, and medicinal herbs.

Perhaps most importantly, I have included a survey of the more serious treatment options for polycystic liver disease. For one out of every five patients, an invasive treatment or surgery may one day be needed to relieve the pain from an enlarged liver. The five major treatments examined here can relieve these symptoms. All can be helpful for particular patients, and all have risks and benefits. This book also surveys the new drugs of potential benefit that are not yet approved for use, but now in clinical trials.

Polycystic Liver Disease includes a glossary of medical terms, a list of informational websites, and an explanation of the liver tests patients may receive. A bibliography of my sources is also included.

Polycystic Liver Disease is information for patients who wish to learn more. It is the author's hope that the information gathered here will be of use to individuals and their families seeking to understand and manage the effects of polycystic liver disease.

-- David Drum

CHAPTER 1
About Polycystic Liver Disease

Polycystic liver disease is a rare disease in which multiple cysts form on or inside the liver. According to the National Institute of Health's Office of Rare Diseases, it affects less than 200,000 people in the United States. The vast majority of people who suffer from polycystic liver disease are women. Most have no bothersome symptoms. Over time, however, a significant minority of patients will develop severe symptoms, making invasive medical treatment necessary.

Most people who have polycystic liver disease are first diagnosed with polycystic kidney disease, one of the most common inherited diseases in the United States and one that affects nearly half a million Americans. Polycystic liver disease was first identified in 1856. In the beginning it was associated with polycystic kidney disease, which manifests in a similar way, as multiple cysts in the kidneys. That polycystic liver disease could occur as a separate disease was only confirmed a century later. When the disease appears without kidney involvement, medical treatments are the same.

In most but not all cases, patients will have cysts on both the kidneys and the liver. According to one study, when polycystic kidney disease is diagnosed, about 30% of those patients also already have polycystic liver disease. By the age of thirty, an estimated 85% of people with polycystic kidney disease will develop cysts on the liver. Generally speaking, people with more advanced polycystic kidney disease also have more numerous liver cysts.

Approximately five percent of the general population has one or more liver cysts and the frequency and size of cysts increases with age. Polycystic liver disease is not fatal. It does not lower life expectancy, and doctors do not consider it life-threatening. Even in people with many liver cysts, the portion of the liver without cysts functions normally.

For most people, polycystic liver disease is diagnosed incidentally, long after cysts have begun to form. More than five cysts on the liver confirm the diagnosis.

A primary care physician may identify the presence of liver cysts by ultrasound or CT scans. An initial work-up by a liver specialist such as a *hepatologist* or a *gastroenterologist* may include a number of tests, and an endoscopic examination of the upper gastrointestinal tract to rule out rare complications such as portal vein hypertension. Ideally, the liver specialist you see will have some experience treating people with polycystic liver disease.

Liver cysts are fluid-filled sacks that can form in any part of the liver. They are round or oval in shape and can be the size of a pinhead, or grow as large as four inches wide. Cysts may be visualized as small water balloons attached to or embedded in the liver, or the liver pictured as something like a bunch of grapes. Liver cysts grow quite slowly. Usually, liver cysts do not adversely affect liver function even in people who also have cystic kidneys. Cysts are typically more numerous and larger in size when they occur in women.

Liver cysts are *not* cancerous. They contain a fluid chemically similar to plasma, that is, a mixture mostly composed of water that includes proteins, salts, hormones, carbon dioxide and other substances.

An estimated four out of five people with liver cysts have no symptoms at all and live with the disease quite well. However, it has been estimated that as many as 20% of patients do have symptoms or complications that may require treatment. Over a period of years, the growth of cysts can enlarge the liver to several times its normal size, sometimes making a woman appear pregnant when she is not.

An enlarged liver creates pressure on other organs in the abdomen and is responsible for symptoms such as pain, shortness of breath, and abdominal distension. As time passes, these symptoms may force a reduction of normal activities and impinge on quality of life. In the most serious cases, the pain and discomfort of symptoms may cause your doctors to recommend one of the surgical treatment options listed in Chapter 6.

Generally speaking, larger and fewer cysts are easier for doctors to manage and treat than smaller cysts which are more numerous. Cysts which appear on the outer surface of the liver are easier to treat than cysts inside the organ, because these are more easily accessed by a surgeon.

Cysts on the pancreas, seminal vesicle, or arachnoid membranes can develop in people with polycystic kidney disease but they are much less common than liver cysts and usually asymptomatic. Pancreatic and arachnoid cysts, for instance, occur in an estimated 8-9 percent of people with polycystic kidney disease, and almost always cause no discomfort.

Some types of liver cysts are not related to polycystic liver disease.

According to the American Liver Foundation, liver cysts may also be caused by the *echinococcus* tapeworm. The parasite is found in animals such as dogs and sheep in various parts of the world including Central and South America and the far western United States.

Choledochal cysts are a congenital condition that usually appears in the first year of life. They result from a genetic disorder called *Caroli's disease* which is characterized by cysts formed in the bile ducts between the liver, the gallbladder, and the intestines. Choledochal cysts are unrelated to polycystic liver disease.

Liver cancer is not a result of liver cysts which are benign by definition.

The risk factors for polycystic liver disease are examined in the next chapter.

CHAPTER 2
What Causes Polycystic Liver Disease?

Mutations in two particular genes are believed to be a factor in polycystic liver disease when it occurs alone. Polycystic kidney disease has also been linked to genetic abnormalities. Researchers have identified several risk factors for polycystic liver disease.

Simply growing older is a risk factor. Liver cysts grow over time and are more common in older people. Although cysts may be detected during adolescence, bothersome symptoms, if they occur, frequently come much later. A great many people diagnosed with polycystic liver disease are in their forties or fifties. In one large study, older women with both polycystic kidney disease and polycystic liver disease had more liver cysts than younger women with both conditions. Another study found liver cysts in 60-75% of patients with polycystic kidney disease who were on dialysis.

A second risk factor is the severity of kidney dysfunction, particularly in patients with mutations in the PKD1 or PKD2 genes linked to polycystic kidney disease. People with more severe kidney cysts and decreased creatinine clearance are more likely to have liver cysts.

Simply being female is a risk factor. Women are much more likely to have polycystic liver disease than men. Some doctors estimate that liver cysts are eight to ten times more common in women than in men. Men with polycystic liver disease are also less likely to develop enlarged livers than women.

Women with polycystic liver disease have the same chance of a successful pregnancy as women without the disease. However, the number of pregnancies can correlate with the number of liver cysts, so women who wish to become pregnant should discuss the effects of a pregnancy with their doctors. Women who have been pregnant more frequently are more likely to have larger or more numerous liver cysts.

Previous use of exogenous estrogens, or estrogens not manufactured inside the body, is a risk factor. Estrogens are female steroid hormones metabolized in the liver and it is noteworthy that estrogen receptors have been identified in the tissue lining liver cysts. A higher incidence of high blood pressure, liver cancer, and increased sulfobromophthalein retention on BSP tests has been reported in women using oral contraceptives or birth control pills. Many experts recommend discontinuing contraception in the form of birth control pills.

Exogenous estrogens are also used in hormone replacement therapy or HRT to relieve the symptoms of menopause. The estrogen used in HRT in the United States, Premarin, is an exogenous estrogen similar but not identical to estrogen produced inside the human body.

HRT can cause liver cysts to increase in size. A 1997 study conducted in Denver looked at two small groups of women with polycystic kidney disease, one group taking HRT and the other group not taking the therapy. Re-examined after one year, researchers found that women on HRT had an average increase of 7% in total liver volume while women not on HRT saw their liver volumes *reduced* by an average of 2%. In the Denver study, women with larger livers experienced more symptoms such as abdominal pain and shortness of breath.

In 2008, a study in Mexico of 42 patients with polycystic liver disease found that women receiving hormone replacement therapy or HRT had more symptoms on diagnosis and required a more frequent use of invasive therapies than postmenopausal women not taking HRT. In the same study, the authors noted that a high alkaline phosphatase level was also more frequently associated with the need for invasive treatment.

The next chapter examines the important role of the liver in the body, a primary concern in polycystic liver disease.

CHAPTER 3
About the Liver

The liver is the largest organ inside the body and one of the most important. Considered the body's "chief of staff" in Traditional Chinese Medicine, the liver is so important to life that it is the only organ inside the body which can regenerate itself. Reddish brown in color, the liver performs more than five hundred metabolic functions needed to maintain good health, and life itself.

Both an organ and a gland, the liver is located inside the abdomen beneath the diaphragm on the right side of the body. It sits atop the stomach, some of the colon, and the right kidney.

Normally about the size of a deflated football, the liver of a healthy adult typically weighs between two and a half and three and a half pounds. The liver contains four lobes and eight segments. It has five ligaments and five fissures, and is covered by a tough fibrous sheath called Glisson's capsule.

The liver has a role in regulating blood volume. It has been estimated that about one-fourth of each person's blood supply passes through the liver every minute. At any one time, more than 10% of the body's blood supply may be found in the liver. The liver is nourished by blood from both arteries and veins with the majority of its blood supply coming from the portal vein.

From the portal vein, the liver receives blood and digested food from the intestinal tract. From this mixture, the liver removes and stores carbohydrates, iron, and vitamins. It manufactures proteins and blood clotting factors. It filters out toxins created during the process of digestion. It cleans the blood of bacteria, alcohol, and drugs. The liver breaks down and regulates certain hormones including sex hormones.

The liver manufactures cholesterol, a major component of bile. It secretes bile into a series of bile ducts that meet at the gall bladder, which is nestled beneath the liver. The gall bladder removes water and shunts concentrated bile back into the small intestine and this helps us digest food, particularly fats.

The liver stores most of the body's reserves of glucose, a vital carbohydrate which can be released as needed for quick energy. The liver stores water soluble Vitamins A, B12, D, E, and K. It handles protein and nitrogen metabolism, and secretes chemicals which help blood clot.

The liver is a source of body heat. It has a major role in fighting infections, too.

The growth of cysts on the liver is the root cause of most common symptoms of polycystic liver disease which are examined in the next chapter.

CHAPTER 4
Symptoms and Complications

P eople with polycystic liver disease can experience a number of symptoms associated with the growth of liver cysts, and the increased size of the liver. While most patients have no significant problems with liver cysts, an estimated 20 percent of patients may develop severe symptoms. Symptoms can be *acute* or sudden. They can also be *chronic* or long-lasting. Complications that may occur such as cyst infection, hemorrhage, and portal vein hypertension are also addressed in this chapter.

THE SYMPTOM OF ACUTE PAIN

The most common acute symptom experienced by people with polycystic liver disease is pain. Pain was reported by almost 37% of patients at diagnosis in a 2005 study. Other reports show pain afflicts as many as 60 percent of patients with an established diagnosis of polycystic kidney disease. Pain can come from the pressure of many cysts, from only a few cysts, or from cysts which press against arteries, veins, or bile ducts. Women who have given birth more than two times more frequently experience acute pain.

In people with both kidney and liver cysts, pain is more likely to stem from liver cysts than kidney cysts. The pain of liver cysts is also more disabling. Dietary strategies such as eating smaller and more frequent meals may help, as can regular moderate exercise, but noninvasive pain control measures do not always completely vanquish pain.

CHRONIC SYMPTOMS

As the liver enlarges, it squeezes and displaces other organs. Over time, the growth of liver cysts can result in uncomfortable chronic or persistent symptoms.

Chronic pain from kidney or liver cysts has been described as a steady persistent pain which is often made more uncomfortable by standing or walking. The pain is frequently localized, that is, the source of the pain can be found with one finger. The most disabling pain is often caused by liver cysts, particularly in women who have had more than one child. Discomfort is often more severe when the body is erect.

The pressure of an enlarging liver is responsible for not only abdominal discomfort but also related chronic symptoms which can occur such as abdominal heaviness or distension, limited mobility, fatigue, shortness of breath, swelling of the extremities or edema, and sometimes continuous or intermittent abdominal or back pain. Abnormalities of the connective tissue such as mitral valve prolapse, intracranial aneurysms or abdominal hernia can occur. The incidence of abdominal hernia is about 10% according to a 2010 report.

Chronic symptoms caused by an enlarged liver include gastrointestinal complaints such as a feeling of "fullness" or early satiety, nausea, and heartburn.

These may be controlled to some extent by diet, that is, by eating smaller and more frequent meals and careful food choices. However, over a prolonged period of time, these symptoms can decrease nutrient intake. When these symptoms are severe, the diet should be evaluated to avoid malnutrition or muscle wasting.

According to a survey of pain management techniques published in *Kidney International,* the most conservative treatments for pain resulting from kidney cysts or liver cysts include physical measures such as ice massage, heating pads, whirlpool baths, and the Alexander postural technique which can sometimes help with lower back pain. Behavior modification techniques are sometimes helpful in managing chronic pain. Mind–body techniques such as meditation may help relieve anxiety and mental distress. Other conservative physical interventions for pain which have no significant side effects include transcutaneous electrical nerve stimulation or TENS, and acupuncture. However, these treatments are more effective on pain from kidney cysts than pain from liver cysts. They may have some effect on mild to moderate pain, but they often do not completely eliminate or cure it.

Pain-relieving drugs – Pain-relieving drugs should be used with great care, and after consultation with a medical doctor. The National Kidney Foundation recommends acetaminophen (Tylenol) as the first analgesic of choice for "occasional use in patients with kidney disease." The American Liver Foundation has warned people not to exceed an intake of 3,000 milligrams of acetaminophen a day "for any prolonged period of time." Acetaminophen is an ingredient in hundreds of over-the-counter medications and also in prescription pain-relievers such as Vicodin; these should be taken into account in calculating a safe dose. The American Liver Foundation cited a study published in the *Journal of the American Medical Association* showing that healthy adults who took the maximum dose of acetaminophen for two weeks showed "drastically increased liver enzyme levels which could lead to liver damage." Another study published in the journal *Hepatology* found that the consistent use of high levels of acetaminophen was associated with several incidences of liver failure. Acetaminophen should not be taken by patients who chronically abuse alcohol, as this can result in liver failure.

As a second-line pain reliever, the study of pain-relieving techniques published in *Kidney International* stated that a non-acetylated salicylate such as salsalate is probably the next safest choice. Non-steroidal anti-inflammatory drugs or NSAIDs such as aspirin are widely taken for minor pain but their use should be limited to a few days by people with kidney or liver insufficiency.

NSAIDs are near the top of the list of drugs that can cause liver injury and they should not be taken long-term. An estimated 10% of the drug-induced liver toxicity in the United States is NSAID-related. "Combination" analgesics often contain NSAIDs and should also be avoided.

In the past, some NSAIDs have been withdrawn from the market due to liver toxicity. One of them, sulindac, is associated with 5-10 times more serious liver reactions than other NSAIDs. Ibuprofen has a very low liver toxicity rate according to one study, although it may increase the risk of liver injury when taken by people with chronic hepatitis C. Cox-2 inhibitors, which are chemically similar to NSAIDs, have caused kidney toxicity in mice and their use should be limited as should the use of stronger pain-relieving drugs such as Tramadol, clonidine, and the opiods.

COMPLICATIONS

In addition to the pressure from an expanded liver, sudden intense acute pain can result from complications such as the infection, hemorrhage, rupture, or torsion of a cyst or cysts.

In a study of 40 Canadians with polycystic liver disease, questioned between one and 15 years after diagnosis, 22% had experienced the complication of cyst bleeding, 12.5% had experienced cyst rupture, and 12.5% had experienced cyst infection. Approximately 30% had required a medical intervention. A large study in Mexico found similar rates of these complications among a group of 41 patients with polycystic liver disease.

Cyst infections are the most dangerous of these complications, because they can lead to sepsis which is potentially life-threatening. Infections can be difficult for a doctor to pinpoint and treat. An initial workup for polycystic liver disease usually includes an analysis of ascetic fluid if present in the abdominal cavity. Fluid can accumulate in the abdomen due to a leakage from the veins or lymph system. If ascetic fluid is present, an analysis of the fluid can rule out a process of infection.

Chills and fever, and often pain in the upper right abdomen, can be symptoms of an infection. Cyst infections can be caused by bacteria or amoebae, but bacterial infections are more common. Liver enzymes are often elevated. Typically, a physician identifies the cause of the infection by a blood culture, by drawing fluid from the suspected cyst to analyze it, or both. An analysis of this helps a doctor determine which drug to use after microorganisms are identified.

To control a cyst infection, traditional first-line antibiotics such as the penicillins, cephalosporins, and aminoglycosides are usually not effective in penetrating kidney or liver cysts, according to the evaluation of pain management techniques published in *Kidney International*. Most experienced doctors utilize an antibiotic or combination of antibiotics which can penetrate cysts such as trimethoprim-sulfamethoxazole, fluoroquinolones, clindamycin, vancomycin, metronidazole, ciprofloxacin, amikacin, or ceftriaxone. Cyst drainage can be done in tandem with antibiotic treatment and employing them both is often the treatment of choice. If appropriate drug treatments fail, after about two weeks, closed drainage of the infected cyst, guided by ultrasound or CT scanning, can be undertaken.

Hemorrhages are much less common than infections, but may be mistaken for infections. Symptoms include pain in the upper right quadrant of the abdomen, and fever. Diagnosis relies on imaging techniques. MRI imaging is currently the best way to differentiate a hemorrhage from an infection. This problem often resolves itself within a week, with bed rest and hydration, but can take several weeks to resolve. Liver cysts can also rupture, possibly causing acute pain and ascites. Cyst ruptures are extremely rare and usually caused by trauma.

Obstructive jaundice is rare in people with polycystic liver disease. It is caused by a blockage of normal bile flow out of the liver by gallstones, inflammation, or trauma. Jaundice causes the skin and eyes to turn yellow and can cause acute abdominal pain and fever.

PORTAL VEIN HYPERTENSION

In the human body, veins carrying blood from the stomach, intestine, spleen, and pancreas merge to form the *portal vein* which supplies approximately 75% of the blood used by the liver. If blood flow from the portal vein to the liver is reduced, blood backs up and creates high blood pressure inside the vein.

Portal vein hypertension is rare, affecting an estimated 2-5% of patients. It is diagnosed by ultrasound or CT scan and in special cases by MRI. Complications of portal vein hypertension can include *ascites,* an accumulation of serous fluid in the abdomen, or bleeding in the related veins. Severe ascites can cause abdominal distension. Portal vein hypertension can also compress bile ducts resulting in an impeded flow of bile.

When blood pressure in the portal vein becomes too high, blood backs up and seeks other ways to flow back to the heart. One place blood can back up is in the veins to the esophagus which can create *esophageal varices*. Mesh tubes called *stents* are sometimes surgically inserted to strengthen or relieve pressure on the portal vein or other blood vessels or ducts.

To maintain good health, the diet and lifestyle issues covered in the next chapter are of great importance.

CHAPTER 5
Diet and Lifestyle

W hat you eat and how you conduct your life are fundamentally important factors in good health. This chapter looks at exercise, nutrition, and lifestyle choices. It also includes a short section on medicinal herbs.

REGULAR EXERCISE

Maintaining a healthy body weight is strongly advised for people with polycystic liver disease, and indeed for all people. Exercise and a well-balanced diet are the keys to maintaining a healthy weight.

Physical activity stimulates the heart, the liver, and other organs by increasing the circulation of blood. Exercise counteracts a feeling of fatigue, combats stress, increases energy levels, and works against depression. It is useful in helping maintain normal body weight, and helps prevent fatty liver disease. One study showed that regular exercise results in increased oxygen consumption and greater strength in patients with viral hepatitis and other chronic liver disorders. In a study of people with polycystic liver disease conducted in Mexico City, researchers noted that overweight patients with a body mass indicator or BMI of greater than 25 had a trend of being susceptible to complications requiring invasive treatment of liver cysts.

If possible, people with polycystic liver disease should consult a registered dietitian or nutritional specialist familiar with the disease. Mayo Clinic registered dietitians Nickie Francisco-Ziller and Sara Di Cecco, MS, recommend daily exercise for people with polycystic liver disease. However, they note that people who suffer from symptoms of fatigue or discomfort often do best with shorter but more frequent exercise sessions. For example, they say, many people might do best with two or three 10-

15 minute walks or sessions on an exercise bike per day, as tolerated.

People who are obese upon diagnosis often benefit from a program of healthy weight reduction, which helps preserve liver function and strengthens overall health. However, standard measurements of overweight or obesity can be skewed for people with late-stage polycystic liver disease. The Mayo Clinic dietitians note that an enlarged liver can artificially inflate both weight and BMI measurements, making patients appear to be overweight on paper when they are actually muscle wasted. For these people, a Subjective Global Assessment or SGA, or strength measurements such as a hand grip dynamometer, are more accurate and useful than BMI in determining nutritional status.

GOOD NUTRITION

For a nutritious diet, minimize your intake of processed foods and junk foods which often contain considerable amounts of added salt, sugar, flavor enhancers, preservatives, and other chemicals. Watch the intake of saturated fat, fried food, or sugary food with empty calories, as directed by your doctor or a nutritional expert. A 2008 study at St. Louis University Liver Center found evidence of liver damage in rats that were fed fast food, but the damage was reversed when rats were switched to a more nutritious diet. Animal studies have found that low fat, low protein diets slow the progression of kidney disease and the growth of liver cysts in lab animals.

Drinking adequate water assists the digestion and elimination process and minimizes the possibility of dehydration. There is theoretical evidence that increasing the normal intake of water might help some people with mild to moderately severe polycystic kidney disease by helping flush toxins out of the body. Clinical trials are being conducted at the Mayo Clinic to test this theory. However, many dietitians recommend drinking only normal amounts of water in the early stages of the disease, and later, when caloric intake is more problematic, consuming beverages containing more calories and nutrients. A little lemon juice in the water may help digestion.

Fresh organic produce is probably easier on the liver than fruits and vegetables which are not organic, since there are no chemical residues on organic produce to be removed by the liver. Organic produce is also not genetically modified. Although a great many scientists consider genetically-modified food crops to be safe, a meta-analysis of 19 studies of genetically modified maize and soybeans, most of which were engineered to contain a pesticide or "tolerate" large amounts of herbicide, found some evidence of kidney and liver damage in mammals. Other studies have turned up evidence of liver damage related to small amounts of chemicals such as lead, mercury, and certain pesticides in foods. Raw or uncooked shellfish should be avoided because of possible contamination by marine toxins or hepatitis A, but well-cooked oysters and clams are fine.

At least five portions of fresh vegetables and fruits per day comprising about one-third of the diet are recommended for most people. Fresh fruits and vegetables are very low in sodium and high in fiber, vitamins, and minerals. Vegetables and fruits can be useful additions to a diet for weight loss. High fiber foods such as vegetables, beans, and fruits bind to bile in the large intestine and carry it out of the body. A study published in the *New England Journal of Medicine* found that vegetarian women excrete more estrogen and have lower levels of estrogen in blood plasma. Vegetables such as legumes and cruciferous vegetables contain phytoestrogens that theoretically block some effects of stronger estrogens made in the body and xenoestrogens which enter the body from meat and farmed fish given steroids to make them gain weight. Interestingly, a study in Poland found that beetroot juice had a protective effect on the livers of lab animals. Another recent study found that the intake of vegetable protein is inversely related to blood pressure. However, Francisco-Ziller and Di Cecco note that the symptom of early satiety sometimes works against the intake of large amounts of fiber for people with polycystic liver disease. If an individual does not have an adequate intake of protein or calories to maintain their nutritional status, they note, he or she may need to actually reduce his or her intake of vegetables such as carrots, celery or lettuce.

According to Medline Plus, a service of the National Institutes of Health, general dietary recommendations for people with chronic liver disease aim at minimizing stress on the liver by restricting the intake of protein and fats, increasing carbohydrate consumption, and supplementing with B complex vitamins.

However, Mayo Clinic dietitians note that polycystic liver disease is different from other chronic liver diseases in that, except for the cysts, the liver is functioning normally. For this reason, they often recommend a well-balanced diet, aiming for a daily intake of protein of between 1-1.2 grams per kilogram dry weight, with no particular restrictions on carbohydrates or fats for most people. For a 150-pound woman (weighing a bit more than 68 kilograms) this would come out to approximately 68 grams or two and a half ounces of protein per day. For purposes of illustration, approximately one ounce of protein may be found in four ounces of cooked salmon, grilled chicken, or mostly lean cooked ground beef.

The Mayo Clinic dietitians recommend slightly more protein than typically recommended for people with other forms of chronic liver disease. Recommendations are also a bit higher than the recommended daily allowance for protein for many people. However, they stress that adequate protein in the diet is vital, since protein helps the body repair damaged cells.

"Patients are more likely to burn muscle mass in times of fasting or stress so they need adequate carbohydrates and protein frequently to offset this," Francisco-Ziller and Di Cecco observe.

For people in the early stages of polycystic liver disease, the dietitians recommend a healthful diet, regular exercise and weight control if needed. In the later stages of the disease, recommendations become more symptom-based. Individuals with symptoms of fullness or early satiety often cannot eat large meals and are typically advised to take small, frequent meals of nutrient-dense, calorie-rich foods in order to maintain their nutritional status. In some cases, dietitians say, nutritional supplement drinks or protein bars may be helpful for these people in achieving their nutritional goals.

After surgical treatments such as a liver resection, according to Francisco-Ziller and De Cecco, the diet will remain similar to the diet before surgery. Adequate calories and protein in small frequent meals will be recommended, particularly during the post-operative period, and nutritional supplement drinks may be required until recovery from surgery is complete. For people who undergo a liver transplant, dietary recommendations are similar but greater care must be taken with food safety and preparation. Among other things, because of drug interactions, grapefruit, pomegranate and Seville oranges and their juice must be permanently avoided after the liver transplant.

Here are some additional thoughts on nutrition:

Protein cannot be stored in the body, unlike carbohydrates and fats. A protein deficiency can lead to malnutrition but too much protein puts stress on the liver. During the process of digestion, the metabolism of proteins releases nitrogen in the form of ammonia, a toxin which must be removed by the liver. An ingredient in many household cleaners and commercial fertilizers, ammonia is created in the body when foods such as meat are digested. In people with more severe forms of chronic liver disease, a buildup of ammonia in the body can cause brain damage. Vegetable protein may be less stressful on the liver than animal protein, but this has not been confirmed for polycystic liver disease.

Carbohydrates burn cleanly in the body, and help in the production of insulin which may help remove toxins. Starchy foods such as pasta, rice, cereal and potatoes provide slow-release energy. Carbohydrates are stored in the liver as glycogen, but a compromised liver may not process and store glycogen in normal amounts.

Fats may help preserve protein in the body and prevent protein breakdown. However, they are digested more slowly than other macronutrients and may delay gastric emptying. Mayo Clinic dietitians do not restrict the consumption of fats in most cases. However, they note, if bilirubin levels are elevated, or if fat intolerance manifests as diarrhea or increased abdominal discomfort after eating fatty foods, fat intake may be restricted. Greasy foods, which are often high in sodium, are sometimes difficult to tolerate for people with liver disease.

Salt (sodium chloride) or sodium is often restricted in people with polycystic liver disease. Most Americans eat far too much salt, an average of 3,400 milligrams per day, according to the Centers for Disease Control (CDC). An estimated 75 percent of Americans' sodium consumption comes from processed or restaurant foods. Excess sodium moves through the liver to the blood and is excreted by the kidneys. CDC dietary guidelines currently call for an intake of less than 1,500 milligrams per day for African-Americans, people over 40, or people with high blood pressure. Too much sodium increases the possibility of infections. In addition to its effects on blood pressure, excessive sodium can contribute to fluid retention, particularly in the form of ascites, or a swelling of the ankles or legs called *edema*. Mayo Clinic dietitians recommend an intake of less than 2,000 milligrams of sodium per day for people with polycystic liver disease but warn that restricting salt intake too severely may compromise necessary protein and carbohydrate intake. As a general rule, many experts advise against adding table salt to foods.

VITAMINS

Vitamin supplements are sometimes be useful in maintaining nutritional status. The liver stores Vitamins A, D, E, K, and zinc. These vitamins are often depleted in people with chronic liver disease but the incidence of nutrient depletion has not been studied in people with polycystic liver disease.

One way to assure an intake of the above nutrients is to include foods in the diet which contain them. According to the National Institutes of Health, foods high in Vitamin A include sweet potatoes baked with peel, beef liver, carrots, and spinach. Foods containing high amounts of Vitamin D (which is made naturally from exposure of the skin to sunlight) include fatty fish such as salmon, tuna and mackerel. Foods high in Vitamin E include wheat germ or safflower oil, sunflower seeds, nuts such as almonds and hazelnuts, and peanut butter. Much Vitamin K is found in green vegetables such as kale, spinach, broccoli, cabbage, and Brussels sprouts. High concentrations of zinc are found in red meat and some seafood such as oysters.

If you are eating a well-balanced diet and maintaining your weight, you probably do not need supplemental vitamins. Mayo Clinic dietitians recommend a multivitamin with 100 percent of US recommended daily allowances for people not eating an adequate and balanced diet which includes a great many of us. However, the *iron content* of multivitamins should be discussed with a medical doctor as some patients have conditions which limit iron intake.

Laboratory tests can uncover deficiencies of particular vitamins. For example, the 25-hydroxy vitamin D test is considered the gold standard test for Vitamin D deficiency. Blood serum tests are available to check levels of Vitamin A, Vitamin K, Vitamin E and zinc. A hair analysis can also be done for mineral deficiencies although some dispute the value of this test. If the patient is deficient in particular vitamins, supplementation may be in order.

In one study, more than 90% of people with chronic liver disease were found to be deficient in Vitamin D. Vitamin D deficiencies are also often found in people with impaired kidney function. The University of Maryland's website states that people with chronic liver disease often have low levels of Vitamin K, which is found in green leafy vegetables and other foods. A Mayo Clinic study published in 2012 found that liver cysts were significantly reduced in rats given a form of Vitamin K. However, since Vitamin K has an effect on blood clotting, Vitamin K supplements can only be prescribed by a medical doctor. Drug-nutrient interactions can occur between Vitamin K and blood thinning medications such as Warfarin (Coumadin). Generally speaking, large quantities of supplemental Vitamin A should be avoided by people with liver problems. Vitamin A is safer in the beta-carotene form.

The abuse of alcohol is known to damage the liver and can trigger additional health problems. Smoking should be avoided, as the toxins in cigarette smoke must be removed by the liver and can cause oxidative stress. Caffeine may promote the growth of cysts, and many doctors recommend that it be avoided. However, Mayo Clinic dietitians note that the evidence for eliminating caffeine from the diet is scanty, and say that a few studies show a benefit for liver health. Francisco-Ziller and Di Cecco suggest you eliminate caffeine if it causes diarrhea or if you are taking medication for high blood pressure.

Of course, always wash your hands before preparing food. Wash fresh produce with running water and friction, that is, by rubbing with the hands or a vegetable brush, to remove chemical residues prior to use.

LIFESTYLE ISSUES

People with chronic liver disease should be very careful with aerosol sprays such as household cleaners, according to the Mayo Clinic website. When using cleaners, make sure the room is well ventilated or wear a mask. Products such as insecticides, herbicides, fungicides, and paint should be avoided or used with great care. As an example of the harm such products may cause, a 2009 study concluded that several different formulations of the herbicide glyphosate (Roundup) disrupted hormone function and killed liver cells even at very low doses.

When you must use such chemicals, protect yourself with a mask and hat, wear long sleeves and other recommended protection, and avoid direct contact with the chemical. Always follow manufacturer's instructions when using chemicals. Chemicals taken into the body by physical contact, eating, or even breathing must ultimately be removed by the liver and kidneys. Vinegar and water, with lemon or soap added, is a natural alternative to commercial products for many housecleaning chores.

MEDICINAL HERBS

Some herbs may have a mild beneficial or protective effect on the liver, but this has only been confirmed in animal studies and not in studies with human subjects. Not all herbs are safe. Some herbs damage the liver and should be avoided. Possible interactions with pharmacological drugs and the lack of standardization in herbal products are other reasons to be cautious in their use.

The herb *milk thistle*, an old folk remedy for liver ailments, is believed to block toxins from entering the liver or to remove them. Milk thistle has a good safety profile, and has shown a benefit in some studies against Hepatitis C, but there is as yet no evidence to support its use in polycystic liver disease. In 2000, a government agency analysis of 16 clinical trials found a small positive protective effect against several liver toxins with milk thistle but concluded that available research did not establish the herb's efficacy.

Dandelion is another folk remedy for liver problems. It is of unproven benefit to people with liver cysts, but probably safe. A study in Korea found that dandelion extract protected against chemically-induced liver damage and oxidative stress in the livers of rats. Another study found dandelion protected against liver toxicity from acetaminophen in mice.

Turmeric or curcumin, another folk remedy, is a spice from India used in curries and other dishes. A 2010, an Austrian study demonstrated reduced liver damage and fibrosis in mice given curcumin.

The herb *schizandra,* an adaptogen employed in Chinese traditional medicine, is believed to support liver and kidney health. A study in Japan found that schizandra cured certain liver injuries in rats.

Cinnamon can lower blood sugar and may have a protective effect on the liver. A study in Egypt found a protective effect on the livers of rats given daily extracts of cinnamon oil for seven days.

Precautions: Some medicinal herbs may *harm* the liver. According to the National Institutes of Health, these include *Kava Kava, pennyroyal*, and *black cohosh. Comfrey* is not recommended for people with liver disease.

Licorice root is sometimes recommended for liver ailments; but according to Medline Plus, licorice can raise blood pressure, lower blood potassium levels, and may act like an estrogen in the body.

Uva ursi is sometimes used to prevent or treat urinary tract or bladder infections or for kidney stones. However, uva ursi can be toxic and should be taken under the supervision of a medical doctor. According to a review on the website of Penn State Hershey Medical Center, hydroquinone, a component of uva ursi, may cause serious liver damage. Uva ursi can interact with lithium, supplements such as Vitamin C and cranberry juice which make the urine more acidic, iron supplements, NSAIDs, and steroidal drugs. Alternative practitioner Dr. Andrew Weil recommends the herb not be taken for more than a few days as long-term use may irritate the liver or cause eye problems or liver damage.

Scattered instances of liver damage have been reported with other herbs including *Jin Bu Huan, germander, chaparral, shark cartilage,* and *mistletoe.* If you are taking prescription medicines, check with your pharmacist for possible drug interactions before taking herbs.

The next chapter looks at the surgical treatments which are often a last resort for people seeking relief from symptoms of polycystic liver disease.

CHAPTER 6
Surgical Treatments

Doctors do not consider polycystic liver disease life-threatening, but the discomfort of symptoms drives many to seek relief through invasive medical treatment or surgery. Depending on the severity of symptoms, invasive treatment may be necessary even if the liver is not drastically enlarged. There are five accepted medical treatments for treating liver cysts:

* Aspiration or draining of cysts

* Nonsurgical treatment with sclerosing agents

* Laparoscopic and open fenestration surgery

* Liver resection and fenestration
* Liver transplantation

One method of assessing the severity of polycystic liver disease is Gigot's classification which is based on computerized tomography (CT) scans. Gigot's type I classification is less than 10 large cysts, type II is diffuse involvement of the functional portion or *parenchyma* of the liver with large remaining areas without cysts, and type III is massive diffuse involvement of the liver parenchyma with only a few areas of normal tissue between cysts. Doctors take assessments such as these into account when recommending a procedure. For instance, with type I patients, laparoscopic fenestration may be the first option recommended. With type II, it may be open fenestration. With type III, in symptomatic cases it may be a liver resection or liver transplant.

The choice of treatment depends on the severity of symptoms, the distribution of liver cysts, and other factors. In one large study published in 2009, the five-year survival rate after cyst fenestration was 90%. Five-year survival after a partial removal of the liver with cyst fenestration was 92%, and five-year survival after a liver transplant was 60%.

Patients who are highly symptomatic but not good candidates for surgery may be candidates for *hepatic artery embolization,* a new and somewhat experimental procedure which can reduce cyst volume by blocking arterial blood flow.

ASPIRATION OR CYST DRAINAGE

Aspiration or draining of liver cysts, guided by ultrasound or computerized tomography (CT) is a simple medical procedure which involves using long needles to drain fluid from cysts.

Cyst aspiration is rarely employed because the cyst or cysts that are temporarily drained usually fill up again, often within weeks, and symptoms return. Percutaneous catheters cannot be placed in the body to drain cysts after the procedure because of the possibility of infection and abscesses which are complicated by secretions from the cyst. A study published in 1991 in the *American Journal of Surgery* found aspiration had a failure rate in 100% of patients as symptoms returned within two years. Other studies have confirmed these unimpressive results.

However, cyst aspiration can be useful in establishing a link between a particular cyst and the symptom of pain. The procedure can provide temporary relief of pain.

NONSURGICAL TREATMENT
WITH SCLEROSING AGENTS

Liver cysts, if there are not too many, may effectively be treated without open surgery. Treatment with sclerosing agents involves a technique, guided by ultrasound, which drains fluid from cysts, then injects ethanol or nearly pure alcohol into them for a brief period of time. Several studies have confirmed the efficacy of this technique on patients with large liver cysts which often shrink or disappear after treatment. The treatment is used with good results on kidney cysts. However, relief is not always permanent.

Vicente Torres, MD, PhD, a noted authority on polycystic liver disease at the Mayo Clinic, in Rochester, Minnesota, believes this procedure works best for deep-seated cysts because the pressure of the liver helps collapse the cysts. In Europe, some doctors also put sandbags over the patient's abdomen for a period of time to help collapse cysts after treatment.

A research study at a Finnish University studied eight patients with liver cysts and symptoms of pain, vomiting, dyspnea and edema of the legs. Cysts were located by CT scan and ultrasound, aspirated by needle, drained, and then injected with 95-99% sterile absolute alcohol or ethanol. Alcohol was left in the cyst for 20 minutes as patients were "rolled" every few minutes to assure the alcohol came into contact with all sides of the cyst before alcohol was withdrawn. In this study, smaller cysts were treated twice and larger cysts were treated three times. Five patients had side effects from the treatment – mostly mild pain and fever, while three patients had no side effects. Blood alcohol levels rose after treatment but subsided. Hemoglobin, hematocrit, liver function, kidney function and clotting factors remained the same after the procedure. No cyst recurrences were found when patients were followed up between 12-32 months later.

In a later study also conducted in Finland, 25 patients with a total of 59 liver cysts were treated in this manner. Some 97% of procedures were technically successful, according to doctors, and there were no recurrences. Eight cysts in six of the patients completely disappeared, while the diameter of the remaining cysts decreased about two-thirds in size. At follow-up approximately four years after the procedure, more than half the patients had no symptoms, and four had reduced pain, but seven of 25 patients had recurring symptoms due to growth of cysts which were not treated. No major complications resulted from the treatment.

Doctors who have used this treatment call it "safe, effective, and minimally invasive" and "the initial treatment of choice for all patients with symptomatic congenital hepatic cysts." Of the surgical methods discussed below, it has the lowest rate of post-surgical complications. A disadvantage of this treatment is that symptoms can recur and cysts can regrow over time

CYST FENESTRATION
OR DEROOFING

Fenestration or *deroofing* surgery involves draining and removal of cysts from the liver. The primary aim of this surgery is to alleviate symptoms such as pain by reducing the size of the liver without compromising liver function. Fenestration is done through conventional open surgery, or with *laparoscopic surgery* using small incisions, instruments, and cameras.

Laparoscopic surgery is the least stressful on the body but open surgery can be more effective for patients with multiple or deep-seated liver cysts. This surgery is also sometimes employed on kidney cysts.

A French study published in the *Annals of Surgery* in 1997 found liver volume reduced between 41-57% at long-term follow up after fenestration. Doctors observed that the technique was most successful for superficial liver cysts and less successful when fenestration of deep-sited cysts was attempted.

Open fenestration is standard surgery. An incision is made in the abdomen, and liver cysts are manually deroofed by a surgical team. The clear sterile fluid inside cysts is allowed to drain freely into the peritoneal cavity. The surgeon removes cyst roofs and walls back to the edge of the liver itself. Cyst walls are then cauterized by Argon laser coagulation which reduces fluid loss from fenestrated cysts. Fenestration of larger exterior cysts allows the surgeon clear, easily visible access to deeply-seated cysts farther inside the liver.

Open fenestration is harder on the body than laparoscopic surgery. Blood loss is generally greater, post-surgical complications are more frequent, and hospital stays are several days longer. However, open fenestration is superior to laparoscopic fenestration in that it allows the surgeon to see and feel cysts during the procedure; this often produces better results with deep-seated cysts. A more complete removal of deep-seated cysts results in a lower rate of cyst recurrence.

Laparoscopic fenestration uses tiny instruments and cameras inserted into the abdomen through small incisions. Cysts are located through ultrasound. Removal is accomplished without open surgery, although open surgery may be required if there are complications such as cysts which cannot be accessed by laparoscopic equipment.

A study in Belgium published in 2001 examined patients treated with either open or laparoscopic fenestration. This study followed 24 patients with congenital liver cysts, about half with single cyst and the balance with multiple cysts including two patients with polycystic liver disease. The Belgian study concluded that "the laparoscopic approach appears to be the gold standard for the treatment of highly symptomatic or complicated simple liver cysts."

A French study of 13 women with multiple cysts published in 1996 found 11 had immediate relief of symptoms after the operation but the women later developed recurrent symptoms. Two underwent additional operations. The French study concluded laparoscopic surgery was not as effective as open surgery or liver resection, and recommended it be employed only on patients with predominantly large cysts.

An Austrian study published about the same time concluded that the laparoscopic technique was less stressful for the patient and had a similar rate of success to open surgery. This study recommended that laparoscopic therapy be the first choice on symptomatic patients because it is less stressful than open surgery.

Still another study at Edinburgh University in Scotland evaluated 38 patients, mostly female, who underwent 48 operations for symptomatic liver cysts. Twenty-three had simple cysts, and 15 had polycystic liver disease. Thirteen of the group had previously been treated with percutaneous cyst aspiration but symptoms returned. Five in 20 patients treated laparoscopically had significant complications after surgery. Five of 14 patients experienced complications after open surgery, mostly from chest infections. In patients with simple cysts, symptoms recurred in 8% of the patients treated laparoscopically and in 29% treated with open surgery after about 41 months. However, in patients with polycystic liver disease, 71% saw return of symptoms after laparoscopic treatment and 20% after open surgery. The 14 patients who received liver resections saw no return of symptoms. Morbidity or further disorders after laparoscopic reroofing were lower than after open deroofing. No fatalities were reported with either technique.

Laparoscopic deroofing is easier on the body and involves shorter hospital stays than open surgery. One advantage of this method is that it can be repeated, where open surgery cannot. It also produces fewer adhesions. Some researchers concluded that laparoscopic deroofing is "usually curative" for simple cysts, but the results are not so predictable in patients with polycystic liver disease because cysts and symptoms can recur. Others believe laparoscopic fenestration should be reserved for patients with one or a few large dominant cysts located on the outside of the liver in anterior segments of the right lobe, or left lateral segments; these are considered the prime candidates with the greatest chance for success.

LIVER RESECTION AND FENESTRATION

Liver resection and fenestration, a more complicated surgery, provides more satisfactory long-term symptom control for people with polycystic liver disease. Liver resection and fenestration removes a portion of the liver and deroofs cysts in the remainder of the liver. Although very large portions of the liver are sometimes removed, and there are frequently complications, the liver will reform after surgery.

Several studies have found liver resection and fenestration to be an effective treatment for polycystic liver disease, with long-lasting positive results. The surgery is most suitable for people with large polycystic livers and many small and medium-sized cysts. In certain patients with massive cyst involvement, liver resection and fenestration is often a better choice than fenestration alone. However, this is major surgery, often with a long recovery period. Most studies have found a mortality rate between zero and 3 percent with this surgery, but in a few studies mortality has been higher. Experts rate the risk of dying from this surgery at about 2.5 percent.

Liver resection and fenestration is presently applicable to more people with polycystic liver disease than is a liver transplant which is also major surgery. However, both liver resection and liver transplantation are complicated and difficult surgical procedures.

Dr. Torres recommends that either liver resection or liver transplant be done in a specialized center where experienced surgeons, hepatologists, and nephrologists are available. A careful evaluation of the hepatic veins is critical, Dr. Torres has noted, since preservation of the veins draining blood from the liver is essential. At least two segments of the liver must be retained.

Typically, in a liver resection, three or four of the liver's eight segments are removed and the remaining cysts fenestrated in open surgery. The size of the liver is typically reduced by about two thirds. Because the polycystic liver is both rigid and oversized, surgeries are difficult and can last between one and five hours. Both the portal and hepatic vein systems must be preserved. The gallbladder is often but not always removed during the surgery. Blood transfusions are often required. Temporary drainage catheters are frequently installed.

After surgery, a hospital stay of at least a week and usually longer is necessary. Within six to eight weeks, the liver usually grows back. Studies have found a variation in the rate of cyst recurrence but most studies have reported very low recurrence rates. In almost all patients, liver volume remains stable after surgery.

Complications are frequent but usually resolve over time. Ascites is the most common complication from this surgery. A mild postoperative ascites related to vein outflow often resolves, but long-lasting post-operative ascites is frequent particularly in people on hemodialysis or suffering severe liver failure. In a Chinese study of liver resection surgeries published in 2008, about 15 percent of patients experienced post-operative ascites, and others experienced complications such as bile leakage, hemorrhage, or pleural effusion. Patients remained in the hospital from one week to two months after surgery, with an average stay of about 16 days. Symptom recurrence was linked to increases in size from deep residual untreated liver cysts. Surgeries were more difficult and complicated in patients who had previously received cyst fenestration surgeries. The authors of this study called resection and fenestration the treatment of choice for polycystic liver disease.

A Mayo Clinic study published in 1995 evaluated 31 patients who underwent liver resection and fenestration. Eighteen patients experienced post-operative complications such as pleural effusions or transient ascites, and one patient died after surgery from intra-cerebral bleeding. Of the 29 patients who were followed up at approximately two and a half years after the surgery, 28 reported an immediate and sustained relief of symptoms and improved quality of life. The study concluded that selected patients with polycystic liver disease could benefit from the surgery.

In Shanghai, China, a study published in 2010 evaluated 33 patients with severe polycystic liver disease who underwent liver resection and fenestration. About 78% of patients experienced some post-surgical complications and in 38% complications were deemed serious. All were all discharged symptom free after the surgery. Followed up an average of about five years later, the vast majority of patients remained improved. Two of 33 patients died of kidney failure, one had a liver transplant, and three saw recurrence of symptoms between approximately four to eight years after the operation, a recurrence rate of about 14%.

Generally speaking, medical centers which do more of these surgeries have lower rates of mortality than medical centers which perform fewer surgeries. This is also true of liver transplant surgery. A study published in 2003 found that the risk of death from liver resection surgery was 40% less at high volume medical centers, defined as those doing more than 10 liver resections per year, versus hospitals doing fewer surgeries. Of approximately 250 American hospitals which did liver resection surgery at the time of the study, only about one in ten was classified as a high-volume medical center.

LIVER TRANSPLANTATION

The first reported liver transplant for polycystic liver disease was done in 1988. Transplants can be of a complete liver, or of liver segments from live or deceased donors. This is the only treatment which completely cures polycystic liver disease. Kidney failure that is secondary to end-stage liver disease is usually reversible after a liver transplant. Combined liver and kidney transplants are also sometimes performed on patients with both polycystic kidney and liver disease.

Potential recipients of donated organs must be evaluated and placed on a waiting list, and a biological "match" must be found. There is often a long wait and grafts must be done quickly if a suitable organ is located.

Liver transplants are risky and have serious side effects, but show good results in patients with many small cysts that cannot be treated by other means. One-year survival rate is about 90%. The risk of death is significant for this procedure and those that survive must take immunosuppressive drugs for life. People who undergo liver transplants require lower levels of immunosuppressive drugs than are required for other solid-organ transplants.

An early study conducted at UCLA of nine patients with polycystic liver disease who received liver transplants saw eight patients survive with "excellent symptomatic relief and improved quality of life in all the surviving patients." Three of the nine patients received combined liver-kidney transplants, and one of nine patients died. The mean hospital stay was 23 days and the mean blood transfusion was 18 units for these patients. Researchers concluded that appropriately selected patients could have "excellent outcomes" with transplantation.

In a 2001 study of liver transplants for polycystic liver disease conducted in Belgium and the United Kingdom, 14 of 16 adult women who underwent liver transplants for small diffuse cysts were cured of polycystic liver disease. The subjects were between 35-56 years old. Five of the women were clinically malnourished, and several had cholestasis or portal hypertension. Most also had polycystic kidney disease, although only one subsequently received a kidney transplant. One of the 16 women died during surgery and another died six years later.

Some of the patients in the Belgian study attempted to reject the transplanted organ, but that was controlled with steroids or a switch in medication. In this study, one patient underwent a kidney transplant four years after the liver transplant. Patient and graft survival were almost 88% at follow up ranging from three months to nine years after transplant.

Transplant surgeries took between 5-8 hours. Woman in the study experienced complications such as biliary stricture, bleeding, and more. Some patients required no blood transfusions, but one required 22 units. All were given immunosuppressive drugs such as cyclosporine, FFK506, and azathioprine to prevent rejection of the transplanted organ. For 90 percent of patients, steroids were discontinued at three months.

The average hospital stay was about 13 days. Investigators found that surgeries were more difficult, with a tendency for more bleeding, in patients who had undergone previous surgeries such as liver resection and fenestration. The patient who died during surgery had undergone several surgeries to reduce the size of her liver prior to the transplant surgery. Patients who required a liver transplant usually did not need a kidney transplant as well. Women quickly returned to a fully active professional and social lifestyle after transplant surgery, researchers said.

Two other studies, both conducted in Germany, looked at patients who received combined liver and kidney transplantation.

A 2006 study in Hanover, Germany, evaluated 36 patients, mostly women, who received liver transplants or combined liver-kidney transplants for polycystic liver disease. Five of these patients died within two months of transplant surgery, a mortality rate of 14%. In a follow up questionnaire given between five months and 14 years after the transplant surgery, 91% of respondents said they felt "better" or "much better," while 9% said they felt "worse" than before the transplant. More than half those queried participated in sports regularly, and most reported an increased interest in sex. In the end, 78% said they would opt for transplantation again, while 17% were undecided and one patient said she would not undergo transplantation again.

A second German study evaluated results for 38 patients who received simultaneous liver and kidney transplants. Patients were between five and 64 years of age. About two-thirds were women. All had polycystic liver disease and several also had cirrhosis of the liver. Fourteen of these patients died, 10 not long after the surgery. At the time of the study, between one and 12 years after transplant surgery, 24 remained alive with good liver function. Five liver and two kidney re-transplantations were performed during the follow-up period. Researchers observed that patients who had been on dialysis for the longest periods of time had lower survival rates.

They also observed that not every patient with polycystic liver disease needs a transplant of both organs, as only about half of patients with autosomal-dominant polycystic kidney disease develop kidney failure. When performed early, they said the combined transplantations were a safe procedure offering long-term palliation of disease.

The United Network for Organ Sharing manages the organ transplant system in the United States by maintaining a database of potential recipients and matching donors with recipients. In Canada, the Canadian Blood Services maintains a Living Donor Paired Exchange Registry. In Europe, the European PH1 Transplantation Study Group maintains similar data.

There are 270 approved organ transplant centers in the U.S. and about two dozen in Canada. A major drawback to transplantation is that the patient must be placed on an organ donor list. Patients with polycystic liver disease, which most doctors do not consider life-threatening, often receive a low priority when it comes to donated organs because their model for end-stage liver disease (MELD) scores are low.

However, the authors of an article on polycystic liver disease published in 2010 in *Digestive Liver Diseases* observed, "Although the development of liver failure in ADPKD is unusual, cystic liver disease is responsible for significant morbidity and accounts for 10% of deaths of ADPKD patients on dialysis."

A study published in the *New England Journal of Medicine* found that liver transplant centers doing fewer than 20 transplants per year had "significantly higher" mortality rates than larger centers, a difference of about 6%. According to the Scientific Registry of Transplant Recipients, as of the end of 2011 the highest volume transplant centers in the U.S. included the University of California Medical Center, San Francisco, California; the University of California at Los Angeles Medical Center of Los Angeles, California; Baylor All Saints Medical Center, Fort Worth, Texas; New York University Medical Center, New York, New York; New York University Medical Center, New York, New York; Baylor University Medical Center, Dallas, Texas; University of Colorado Hospital/Health Science Center, Aurora, Colorado; Stanford University Medical Center, Stanford,

California; California Pacific Medical Center, San Francisco, California; Hospital of the University of Pennsylvania, Philadelphia, Pennsylvania; Cedars-Sinai Medical Center, Los Angeles, California; and the Mayo Clinic (Rochester Methodist Hospital), Rochester, Minnesota.

HEPATIC ARTERY EMBOLIZATION

A different form of treatment, *transcatheter hepatic artery embolization*, is being studied in Asia, and some centers are preparing to try it in North America. The treatment uses X-ray guidance to insert intravascular coils or polyvinyl alcohol particles into arteries providing blood to particular segments of the liver. Arteries provide most of the blood supply to liver cysts and blocking particular arteries decreases blood flow and reduces the size of the affected segment of the liver.

In Kanagawa, Japan, 30 patients with polycystic liver disease, most already on dialysis because of kidney failure, were treated with transcatheter artery embolization. Pain and fever experienced by patients after the treatment resolved within five days. Followed up from 18-37 months after therapy, 29 patients saw both reduced liver volume and reduced cyst volume as a result of the treatment, although one person in the study experienced increases in both. Average reduction in liver size was 22 percent. No serious complications were reported, and quality of life was improved in almost all patients.

In another trial published in the *Journal of Korean Medical Science*, researchers used hepatic artery embolization techniques developed to treat liver cancer to reduce liver cyst size in four patients with polycystic liver disease. Arteries supplying the dominant segments were blocked using polyvinyl alcohol particles and micro-coils. Two of three patients followed up a year after treatment saw liver and cyst volume substantially decreased. Adverse events reported were fever, pain, nausea, and vomiting. Researchers in Korea concluded that the technique could be a safe, effective option for patients with polycystic kidney disease and liver pain who are not candidates for surgical treatment.

A Chinese study published in 2013 used a mixture of N-butyl-2-cyanoacrylate (NBCA) tissue glue and iodized oil to block selected arteries in 21 patients with massive symptomatic polycystic liver disease. This technique achieved symptom relief in 87% of patients, and resulted in significant decreases in liver and cyst volume after the procedure.

While the medical treatments listed in this chapter are presently the gold standard for treating painful chronic symptoms, the pharmacological drugs listed in the next chapter may hold a promise for future treatments.

CHAPTER 7
Drug Treatments

There are as yet no drugs approved to treat polycystic liver disease, although a few somewhat promising drugs that reduce liver size are now being evaluated in clinical trials.

A long-lasting analogue of somatostatin called *octreotide* is being studied for its effects on polycystic liver disease. The drug is injected once every 28 days by a health care professional. Octreotide targets the cholangiocyte cells which proliferate and secrete fluid to form liver cysts.

A small Italian study published in 2010 evaluated 12 patients treated with octreotide every 28 days over a six-month period. Doctors reported that the drug limited kidney volume growth more than placebo.

Total liver volumes also decreased in patients receiving the drug but remained stable in patients receiving placebo, although there were wide variations in efficacy. Few complications were reported during the time of the study.

An earlier study of octreotide found 22–60% reductions in liver weight, cyst volume, hepatic fibrosis, and mitotic indices in PCK rats. Similar reductions in kidney size were observed in research animals.

Clinical trials utilizing octreotide are currently underway at the Mayo Clinic.

A similar drug called *lanreotide*, another analogue of somatostatin, is also in clinical trials. A six month double blind clinical trial in the Netherlands utilizing lanreotide administered every 28 days saw subjects' liver volume reduced 2.9% in the group receiving lanreotide, while the placebo group saw liver volume increases of 1.6%.

Another somatostatin analog, *pasireotide*, is also in clinical trials.

In an animal study involving PK2 mice, liver cyst growth was blocked by vascular endothelial growth factor inhibition which slowed the proliferation of liver cyst fluid. Inhibiting the epithelial cells which line cysts may open another promising avenue for future research.

APPENDIX A

MEDICAL AND LABORATORY TESTS

This section explains some of the medical tests you may encounter including imaging tests, liver enzyme tests, and liver function tests.

Imaging tests

Several procedures create images or pictures of your liver which are useful to your doctor.

Ultrasound utilizes sound waves to "map" the interior of the body and to detect the location of cysts.

CT or computed tomography scans utilize X-rays processed in a computer to provide interior images of "slices" of the body.

MRI imaging utilizes magnetic imagery to provide a highly detailed "cross section" of the body including the liver and internal organs.

A special X-ray of the kidney called an *intravenous pyelogram* utilizes an injected dye that can be used to diagnose polycystic liver disease.

Liver enzyme and liver function tests

Liver enzyme tests are blood tests that doctors use to detect inflammation and damage to the liver. Liver enzyme tests include the ALT, AST, and alkaline phosphatase tests. *Liver function tests* check how well the liver is working. Liver function tests include the PT, INR, albumin, and bilirubin tests.

Liver enzyme tests:

ALT and AST

The cells in the liver contain proteins called *enzymes* that drive chemical reactions to metabolize nutrients, detoxify harmful substances, make blood clotting proteins, and perform many other vital functions. If ALT and AST are detected together in elevated amounts in the blood, liver damage is most likely present.

ALT and AST are the two main liver enzymes. *Aspartate aminotransferase* (AST), formerly called SGOT, is an enzyme is found in the liver, muscles and many other tissues. *Alanine aminotransferase* (ALT), formerly called SGPT, is an enzyme found almost exclusively in the liver.

The liver filters and processes blood that circulates through the body. When liver cells are damaged or destroyed, enzymes in the cells leak out into the blood, where they can be measured by blood tests. A normal test result for ALT is 7 to 55 units per liter, and for AST a normal result is 8 to 48 units per liter.

Alkaline Phosphatase, 5' Nucleotidase, and GGT

One of the liver's functions is the production of bile, which is returned to the intestine to help digest fats. Bile flows from the liver via a system of small tubes (ducts), and is eventually stored in the gallbladder, under the liver. When the flow of bile is slowed or blocked, blood levels of three liver enzymes rise -- *Alkaline phosphatase (ALP), 5' nucleotidase,* and *Gamma-glutamyl transpeptidase (GGT).* All are checked via blood tests.

Alkaline phosphatase is by far the most commonly tested of the three. ALP is made mostly in the liver. The liver makes more ALP than the other organs or the bones. Damaged liver cells and other conditions cause large amounts of ALP to accumulate in the blood. An ALP test checks for liver disease or damage to the liver. If the ALP level is high, more tests may be done to find the cause. The ALP test may also be used to check the condition of the liver when medicines that might damage the liver are taken. Normal blood test results for ALP range from 45 to 115 units per liter.

If alkaline phosphatase and/or 5' nucleotidase and GGT are elevated, a problem with bile flow is most likely present. Problems with bile flow may be from a problem in the liver, the gallbladder, or the connecting ducts. Normal GGT ranges from 9 to 48 units per liter.

Liver Function Tests:

PT and INR

One function of the liver is to make proteins that are essential to normal blood clotting. True liver function tests check the liver's ability to make these proteins.

Prothrombin time (PT) is a test of the time it takes for a blood sample to clot, under specific conditions in a lab. If low levels of clotting factors are present, the prothrombin time is longer. *International normalized ratio* (INR) is a standardized way for all labs to report PT, so that results from different testing laboratories can be accurately compared.

PT and INR are elevated in people with severe liver disease because the liver does not make normal amounts of certain clotting factors. An elevated PT does not exclusively indicate liver disease and may have other causes related to medication or Vitamin K levels.

PT is often checked together with Partial Thromboplastin Time or PTT, which is not a liver function test. If PT and/or PTT are elevated, a problem with bleeding or blood clotting may be present. Normal PT is 9.5 to 13.8 seconds.

Albumin

Albumin is an essential water-soluble protein made in the liver. It circulates in blood. Albumin levels are low in people with severe chronic liver disease, because the liver does not make normal amounts of albumin. A low level of albumin in the blood is often temporary, so it is not a reliable way to diagnose liver disease. Normal albumin is 3.5 to 5 grams per deciliter.

Bilirubin

When red blood cells break down, a waste product called Bilirubin is created. Bilirubin is processed in the liver and flows from the liver through the bile ducts. Dissolved in bile, bilirubin is excreted in the stool.

In the blood, Bilirubin levels may be elevated in people with impaired bile flow. This can occur in severe liver disease, gallbladder disease, or other bile system conditions. Very high bilirubin levels cause *jaundice,* in which the skin and whites of the eyes turn yellow. Bilirubin can be a useful liver function test in people with a known bile flow problem. An elevated bilirubin may be present in people with hemolytic anemia. Bilirubin may also be detected in the urine. Normal Bilirubin is 0.1 to 1.0 mg/dL.

BSP Test

The BSP or *sodium sulfobromophthalein (Bromsulphalein)* test in the nonjaundiced patient is considered one of the best and most sensitive indicators of liver dysfunction.

Bromosulphalein dye is injected intravenously, at a rate of 5 mg of dye per kilogram of body weight. Within 30-45 minutes, most of the dye is taken up by the liver cells where it is stored, conjugated, and finally excreted in bile. An abnormal retention of sulfobromophthalein represents a disturbance of one or more of these functions.

Decreased blood flow to the liver will also lead to an increased retention of the dye.

APPENDIX B

A GLOSSARY OF MEDICAL TERMS

Autosomal Dominant Polycystic Liver Disease (ADPLD) is polycystic liver disease not accompanied by polycystic kidney disease. It is believed to be caused by mutations in the PRKCSH or SEC63 genes, and perhaps others.

Autosomal Dominant Polycystic Kidney Disease (ADPKD) usually includes genetic abnormalities of the PK1 or PK2 genes, and multiple cysts on both the liver and kidneys.

Ascites -- an accumulation of serous fluid inside the abdomen or peritoneal cavity which houses the liver and other internal organs.

Albumin -- an essential protein, manufactured in the liver, which circulates in the blood.

Allograft or graft -- refers to the transplant of liver or organ tissue from one person to another.

Bile -- a yellow-green fluid produced by the liver which is stored in the gallbladder and released into the intestine to aid digestion.

Bilirubin -- a waste product removed by the liver. It is created when red cells break down.

Bowel – another name for the intestine or gut which runs from the stomach to the anus. The bowel contains two main sections, (1) the small intestine where food is broken down and absorbed and (2) the large intestine which receives the processed food, absorbs water and salt, and forms solid waste.

Cholecystectomy -- a removal of the gallbladder.

Cholelithiasis -- the presence of gallstones.

Choledocolithiasis -- a gallstone in the bile duct.

Cholesterol -- a steroid made in the liver. Cholesterol is essential in making bile, Vitamin D, progesterone, estrogens, testosterone and other hormones.

Cirrhosis -- a chronic disorder of the liver in which fibrous tissue and nodules replace normal tissue, interfering with the flow of blood and normal liver function.

Dietitian – a professional trained in the science of foods and the therapeutic management of diet.

Endoscope – a medical device consisting of a tube, small camera and light used to view the inside of a patient's body in a minimally-invasive procedure.

Enzymes -- complex proteins which trigger or accelerate chemical reactions in the body but remain unchanged themselves, such as the enzymes which help digest food. Liver enzymes assist with chemical reactions in the liver. Elevated levels of the liver enzymes ALT, ALP, AST, GGT and LDH may indicate a liver or bile duct disorder.

Gallbladder –– a muscular sac attached beneath the right lobe of the liver which stores and concentrates bile, then releases it into the intestines to help digest fats.

Gastroenterologist –– a medical doctor who specializes in diseases of the gastronomical tract which include the stomach, esophagus, pancreas, intestines, gallbladder and liver.

Glycogen –– a form of glucose or simple sugar stored in the liver and the muscles. Glycogen is easily changed back to glucose when the body needs quick energy.

Hematologist –– a medical doctor who specializes in conditions that involve the blood.

Hematuria – blood in the urine.

Hemochromatosis -- a genetic disorder in which the body accumulates more iron than needed causing a buildup of iron in tissues and organs. An accumulation of iron creates a "bronze" look to skin pigmentation. Hemochromatosis can lead to liver failure.

Hepatic -- an adjective, having to do with the liver.

Hepatologist -- a medical doctor specializing in the liver.

Hepatic artery – a large short blood vessel that carries oxygen-laden blood directly from the heart to the liver.

Hepatomegaly -- a swelling of the liver beyond its normal size.

Hepatitis -- a viral inflammation of the liver. Five forms of hepatitis have been identified, the most serious of which is Hepatitis C.

Hypercoagulable -- when the body over-produces blood clots due to malfunctions of clotting factors produced in the liver.

Hypertension -- high blood pressure.

Inferior vena cava – the large vein that carries blood back to the heart from the lower part of the body.

Jaundice -- a yellowing of the whites of the eyes or skin caused by a buildup of bile in the body.

Laparoscopic surgery -- a modern surgical technique in which operations in the abdomen are performed through very small incisions using tubes and tiny cameras. Also called *minimally invasive surgery, band-aid surgery,* or *keyhole surgery.*

Nephrologist -- a medical doctor and kidney specialist.

Parenchyma – the essential or functional part of an organ as distinguished from its connective tissue, blood vessels, etc.

Portal vein -- a large vein carrying blood from the stomach, intestine, spleen, and pancreas to the liver.

Portal hypertension -- a condition of elevated blood pressure in the major vein in the liver. Over time, this can seriously damage the liver, and lead to liver failure.

Renal -- an adjective, having to do with the kidneys.

Stent -- a small tube made of plastic or expandable wire mesh that goes inside a blood vessel or duct or bowel to strengthen it or keep it open. A *biliary stent* is used to keep a bile duct open. Stents may be removed.

Symptom – any perceptible change in the body, or functions of the body, which indicates disease. For instance, pain can be a symptom of polycystic liver disease.

Toxin -- chemicals or other waste products that can be harmful to the body when the liver is not filtering the blood correctly.

Varices -- A type of swollen or varicose vein that can appear in veins lining the esophagus and upper stomach when these veins fill with blood and swell due to an increase in blood pressure in the portal vein.

APPENDIX C
Internet Resources

A great deal of information is available on the Internet. Links to web sites of possible interest are listed below.

*

National Library of Medicine
www.nlm.nih.gov/medlineplus/healthtopics.html

*

National Institute of Diabetes and Digestive and Kidney Diseases
www.niddk.nih.gov

*

American College of Gastroenterology
http://gi.org/

*

American Liver Foundation
www.liverfoundation.org
*

American Liver Foundation – Information for patients and families
http://www.liverfoundation.org/patients/
*

Canadian Liver Foundation
www.liver.ca
*

British Liver Trust
www.british**liver**trust.org**.uk**
*

National Liver Foundation (India)
www.nlfindia.com
*

Children's Liver Association for Support Services
www.classkids.org
*

NIH Clinical Trials database
http://clinicaltrials.gov
*

United Network for Organ Sharing
www.unos.org/
*

Canadian Blood Services – Living Donor Paired
Exchange
www.blood.ca/organsandtissues
*

Scientific Registry of Organ Transplants
http://www.srtr.org/
*

European Society for Organ Transplantation
(ESOT)
www.esot.org
*

Genetic and Rare Diseases Information Center
http://rarediseases.info.nih.gov/GARD/AboutGARD
.aspx
*

American Association for the Study of Liver
Diseases
http://www.aasld.org/Pages/Default.aspx
*

Liver Families – Pediatric Liver Disease
http://www.liverfamilies.net/
*

National Organization for Rare Disorders
http://www.rarediseases.org/
*

Online Medical dictionary from National Library of Medicine
www.nlm.nih.gov/medlineplus/mplusdictionary.html
*

Academy of Nutrition and Dietetics (registered dietitians)
www.eatright.org
*

Mayo Clinic information
www.mayo.edu
*

PKDIET
www.pkdiet.com
*

National Kidney Disease Education Program

www.nkdep.nih.gov

*

PKD Foundation
www.pkdcure.org

*

National Kidney Foundation
www.kidney.org

*

American Kidney Fund
www.akfinc.org

*

American Association of Kidney Patients
www.aakp.org

*

Online checker for drug interactions
www.drugs.com/drug_interactions.php

BIBLIOGRAPHY

Chapter 1

Abu-Wasel, B, et al, "Pathophysiology, epideiology, classification and treatment options for polycystic liver diseases," *World J Gastroenterol.* 2013 September 21;19(35):5775-5786.

Basar O, et al, "Recurrent pancreatitis in a patient with autosomal-dominant polycystic kidney disease," *Pancreatology.* 2006;6:160-2.

Chapman AB, "Cystic disease in women: clinical characteristics and medical management," *Adv Ren Replace Ther.* 2003 Jan;10(1)24-30.

Everson GT, et al, "Management of polycystic liver disease," *Curr Gastroenterol Rep.* 2005 Feb;7(1):19-25.

Onori P, et al, "Polycystic liver diseases," *Dig Liver Dis* 2010 April;42(4):261-271. Doi:10.1016/j.dld.2012.01.006.

Russell RT, et al, "Surgical management of polycystic liver disease," *World J Gastroenterol* 2007 October 14;13(38):5052-5059.

Chapter 2

Barahona-Garrido J, et al, "Factors that influence outcome in non-invasive and invasive treatment in polycystic liver disease patients," *World J Gastroenterol.* 2008 May 28; 14(20);3195-3200.

Gabow PA, et al, "Risk factors for the development of hepatic cysts in autosomal dominant polycystic kidney disease," *Hepatology.* 1990 Jun;11(6):1033-7.

Sherstha R, et al, "Postmenopausal estrogen therapy selectively stimulates hepatic enlargement in women with autosomal dominant polycystic kidney disease," *Hepatology.* 1997 Nov. 26(5):1282-6.

Chapter 4

American Liver Foundation, "The American Liver Foundation Issues Warning on Dangers of Excess Acetaminophen," press release issued New York, July 18, 2006.

Bajwa ZH, et al, "Pain Management in Polycystic kidney disease," *Kidney International*, Vol. 60 (2001), pp. 1631-1644.

Bistritz L, et al, "Polycystic liver disease: experience at a teaching hospital," *Am J Gastroenterol*, 2005 Oct;100(10)2212-7.

Bessone F, "Non-steroidal anti-inflammatory drugs. What is the actual risk of liver damage?" *World J Gastroenterol.* 2010 December 7;16(45):5651-5661.

Chaveau D, et al, "Liver Involvement in Autosomal-Dominant Polycystic Kidney Disease: Therapeutic Dilemma," *J Am Soc Nephrol.* 11: 1767-1775 2000.

Donovan AJ, et al, "Hepatic abscess," *World J Surg.* 1991 Mar-Apr;15(2);162-9.

Harris PC, Torres VE, "Polycystic Kidney Disease, Autosomal Dominant." 2002 Jan 10 [Updated

2011 Dec 8]. In: Pagon RA, Bird TD, Dolan CR, et al., editors. *GeneReviews™* [Internet]. Seattle (WA): University of Washington, Seattle; 1993-. Available from: http://www.ncbi.nlm.nih.gov/books/NBK1246/

Larson, A M, et al, "Acetaminophen-Induced Acute Liver Failaure: Results of a United States Multicenter, Prospective Study," *Hepatology* December 2005 DOI 10.1002/hep.20948

Pirson Y, "Extrarenal manifestations of autosomal dominant polycystic kidney disease," *Anv Chronic Kidney Dis* 2010 Mar;17(2):173-80. Doi: 10.1053/j.ackd.2010.01.003.

Telenti A, et al, "Hepatic cyst infection in autosomal dominant polycystic kidney disease," *Mayo Clin Proc.* 1990 Jul;65(7):933-42.

Zahid H B, et al, "Pain management in polycystic kidney disease," *Kidney International*, Vol. 60 (2001) pp. 1631-1644.

Chapter 5

Baghdasaryan A, et al, "Curcumin improves sclerosing cholangitis in Mdr2-/- mice by inhibition of cholangiocyte inflammatory response and portal myofibroblast proliferation," *Gut.* 2010 Apr; 59(4):521-30.

Bankovic-Calic N, et al, "Effect of a modified low protein and low fat diet on histologic changes and metabolism in kidneys in an experimental model of polycystic kidney disease," *Arp Ath Celok Lek.* 2002 Jul-Aug;130(7-8):251-7.

Colle E, et al, "Antioxidant properties of *Taraxacum officinales* leaf extract are involved in the protective effect against hepatoxicity induced by acetaminophen in mice," *J Med Food.* 2012 Jun;15(6):549-56. Soi: 10.1089/jmf.2011.0282.

Elliott P, et al, "Association Between Protein Intake and Blood Pressure," *Arch Intern Med.* 2006;166(1):79-87. Doi:10.1001/archinta.166.1.79.

Francisco-Ziller, Nickie, RD, and Sara Di Cecco, RD, MS, of the Mayo Clinic, Rochester, Minnesota, personal interview and correspondence with author 2013.

Gasniera C, et al, "Glyphosate-based herbicides are toxic and endocrine disruptors in human cell lines." 2009 Toxicology doi:10.1016/j.tox.2009.06.006

Goldin BR, et al, "Estrogen excretion patterns and plasma levels in vegetarian and omnivorous women," *N Engl J Med* 1982 Dec 16;307(25):1542-7.

Krajka-Kuzniak V, et al, "Beetroot juice protects against N-nitrosodiethylamine-induced liver injury in rats," *Food Chem Toxicol.* 2012 Jun;50(6);2027-33.

Lawrence V, et al, "Milk Thistle: Effects on Liver Disease and Cirrhosis and Clinical Adverse Effects" *Evidence Reports/Technology Assessments, No. 21.* Rockville (MD): Agency for Healthcare Research and Quality (US); October 2000. Report No.: 01-E025.

Loguericio C, et al, "Silybin and the liver: From basic research to clinical practice," *World J Gastroenterol.* 2011 May 14; 17(18):2288-2301

Masyuk TV, et al, "Inhibition of Cdc25A suppresses hepato-renal cystogenesis in rodent models of polycystic kidney and liver disease," *Gastroenterology.* 2012 Mar; 142(3):622-633.e4. doi: 10.1053/j.gastro.2011.11.036. Epub2011 Dec 7.

Moselhy SS, et al, "Hepatoprotective effect of cinnamon extracts against carbon tetrachloride induced oxidative stress and liver injury in rats," *Biol Res.* 2009;42(1)93-8. Epub 2009 Jan.

National Institutes of Health Fact Sheets on Vitamins and minerals. ods.od.nih.gov/factsheets/list-VitaminsMinerals

Park CM, et al, "Amelioration of oxidative stress by dandelion extract through CYP2E1 suppression against acute liver injury induced by carbon tetrachloride in Sprague-Dawley rats," *Phytother Res.* 2010 Sep; 24(9):1347-53. Doi: 10.1002/ptr.3121.

Penn State Hershey Medical Center, "Uva ursi," http://pennstatehershey.adam.com/content.aspx?productId=107&pid=33&gid=000278

Pour PM, et al, "Effect of dietary protein on N-nitrosobis (2-oxopropyl) amine-induced carcinogenesis and on spontaneous diseases in Syrian golden hamsters," *J Natl Cancer Inst.* 1986 Jan;76(1)67-72.

Ritland S, "Exercise and liver disease," *Sports Med.* 1988 Aug;6(2):121-6.

Salt Intake Widget, US Centers for Disease Control. www.cdc.gov/widgets/SaltIntake/alt/

Seralini G-E, et al, "Genetically modified crops safety assessment: present limits and possible improvements," *Environmental Sciences Europe.* 2011, 23:10.

Takeda S, et al, "Pharmacological studies on schizandra fruits. III. Effects of wuweizisu C, a lignin component of schizandra fruits, on experimental liver injuries in rats," *Nihon Yakurigaku Zasshi* 1985 Mar; 85(3):193-208.

Torres V, et al, "A Case for Water in the Treatment of Polycystic Kidney Disease," *Clin J Am Soc Nephrol* 4: 1140-1150, 2009.doi:10.2215/CJN.00790209.

Weil, Dr. Andrew, "Uva Ursi," https://www.drweil.com/vitamins-supplements-herbs/herbs/uva-ursi/

"25-hydroxy vitamin D test," MedlinePlus Medical Encyclopedia.

Chapter 6

Becker T, et al, "Results of combined and sequential liver-kidney transplantation." *Liver Transpl.* 2003;9:1067–1078.

Chauveau D, et al, "Liver involvement in autosomal-dominant polycystic kidney disease: therapeutic dilemma," *J Am Soc Nephrol.* 2000; 11: 1767-1775.

Dimick J B, et al, "Hepatic Resection in the United States," *Arch Surg.* Vol 138 Feb. 2003.

Edwards E B, et al, "The Effect of the Volume of Procedures At Transplantation Centers on Mortality after Liver Transplantation," *N Engl J Med* 1999; 341:2049-2053.

Gigot, J-F, et al, "Adult Polycystic Liver Disease: Is Fenestration the Most Adequate Operation for Long-Term Management?" *Annals of Surgery.* 1997; Vol. 225, No. 3 286-294.

Kabbej M, et al, "Laparoscopic fenestration in polycystic liver disease," *Br J Surg.* 1996;83:1697–1701.

Kairaluoma MI, et al. "Percutaneous aspiration and alcohol sclerotherapy for symptomatic hepatic cysts. An alternative to surgical intervention," *Ann Surg.* 1989;210:208–215.

Koperna T, et al. "Nonparasitic cysts of the liver: results and options of surgical treatment," *World J Surg.* 1997;21:850–854; discussion 854-855.

Kirchner GI, et al. "Outcome and quality of life in patients with polycystic liver disease after liver or combined liver-kidney transplantation," *Liver Transpl.* 2006;12:1268–1277.

Lin TY, et al. "Treatment of non-parasitic cystic disease of the liver: a new approach to therapy with polycystic liver,"*Ann Surg.* 1968;168:921–927.

Macedo F I, "Current management of infectious hepatic cystic lesions: A review of the literature," *World J Hepatol.* 2013 September 27;5(9):462-469.

Martin IJ, et al, "Tailoring the management of nonparasitic liver cysts," *Ann Surg.* 1998;228:167–172.

Morino M, et al."Laparoscopic management of symptomatic nonparasitic cysts of the liver. Indications and results," *Ann Surg.* 1994;219:157–164.

Onori P, et al, "Polycystic liver diseases," *Dig Liver Dis.* 2010 April; 42(4):261-271.

Park H C, et al, "Transcatheter Arterial Embolization Therapy for a Massive Polycystic Liver in Autosomal Dominant Polycystic Kidney Disease Patients," *J Korean Med Sci.* 2009 February, 24(1) 57-61.

Pirenne J, et al, "Liver transplantation for polycystic liver disease," *Liver Transpl.* 2001;7:238-245.

Que F, et al, "Liver resection and cyst fenestration in the treatment of severe polycystic liver disease," *Gastroenterology.* 1995;108:487-494.

Russell RT, Pinson CW. "Surgical management of polycystic liver disease," *World J Gastroenterol.* 2007 Oct 14; 13 (38) 5052-9.

Sanchez H, et al, "Surgical management of nonparasitic cystic liver disease," *Am J Surg.* 1991;161:113-118; discussion 118-119.

Schnelldorfer T, et al, "Polycystic Liver disease: A Critical Appraisal of Hepatic Resection, Cyst Fenestration, and liver Transplantation," *Ann Surg.* 2009;250:112-8.

Swenson K, et al, "Liver transplantation for adult polycystic liver disease," *Hepatology.* 1998 Aug;28(2):412-5.

Takei R, et al, "Percutaneous transcatheter hepatic artery embolization for liver cysts in autosomal dominant polycystic kidney disease," *Am J Kidney Dis.* 2007 Jun;49(6):744-52.

Tikkakoski T, et al, "Treatment of symptomatic congenital hepatic cysts with single-session percutaneous drainage and ethanol sclerosis: technique and outcome," *J Vasc Interv Radiol.* 1996;7:235–239.

Torres VE, "Treatment of Polycystic Liver Disease; One Size Does Not Fit All," *Am J Kidney Dis.* 49, 6(June), 2007:725-728.

Tuan-Jie Li, et al, "Treatment of polycystic liver disease with resection-fenestration and a new classification," *World J Gastroenterol.* 2008; 14(32) 5066-5072.

Turnage RH, et al, "Therapeutic dilemmas in patients with symptomatic polycystic liver disease,"*Am Surg.* 1988;54:365–372.

van Erpecum KJ, et al, "Highly symptomatic adult polycystic disease of the liver. A report of fifteen cases," *J Hepatol.* 1987;5:109–117.

Vauthey JN, et al, "Adult polycystic disease of the liver," *Br J Surg.* 1991;78:524–527.

Vons C, et al, "[Liver resection in patients with polycystic liver disease," *Gastroenterol Clin Biol.* 1998;22:50–54.

Wang MQ, et al, "Treatment of symptomatic polycystic liver disease: transcatheter super-selected hepatic arterial embolization using a mixture of NBCA and iodized oil," *Abdom Imaging.* 2013 Jun;38(3):465-73. Doi: 10.1007/s00261-012-993-1.

Yang GS, et al, "Combined hepatic resection with fenestration for highly symptomatic polycystic liver disease: A report on seven patients," *World J Gastroenterol.* 2004;10:2598–2601.

Chapter 7

Amura CR, et al, "VEGF receptor inhibition blocks liver cyst growth in pkd2 (WS25/-) mice," *Am J Physiol Cell Physiol.* 2007 Jul;293(1):C419-28. Epub 2007 May 2.

Caroli A, et al, "Reducing polycystic liver volume in ADPKD: effects of somatostatin analogue octreotide," *Clin J Am Soc Nephrol.* 2010 May;5(5):783-9. Epub 2012 Feb 25.

Masyuk TV, et al, "Octreotide inhibits hepatic cystogenesis in a rodent model of polycystic liver disease by reducing cholangiocyte adenosine 3',5'-cyclic monophosphate. *Gastroenterology.* 2007 Mar;132(3):1104-16. Epub 2006 Dec 20.

Van Keimpema L, et al, "Lanreotide reduces the volume of polycystic liver: a randomized, double-blind, placebo-controlled trial," *Gastroenterology.* 2009 Nov; 137(5):1661-8.e1-2 Epub 2009 Jul 29.

ABOUT THE AUTHOR

D avid Drum is a medical journalist based in Los Angeles. He is the author or co-author of seven nonfiction books in the health area, and more than one thousand magazine articles and other works of writing.

David Drum's health books are useful and well-organized. They utilize an honest, educational, common sense approach and are known for their well-researched content and for their presentation of factual information in an empathetic, patient-centered, compassionate tone of voice.

The author has been a newspaper reporter, a teacher, an advertising copywriter, and a contributing editor and correspondent for newspapers, trade magazines and wire services. He has been working as an independent journalist and author since 1978. In addition to this book, others written or co-written by David Drum include:

-- *The Type 2 Diabetes Source-book*, 3rd Edition, McGraw-Hill, 2006, co-written with Terry Zierenberg, RN, CDE

--*What Your Doctor Might* Not *Tell You About Uterine Fibroids*, Warnerbooks, 2003, co-written with Scott Goodwin, MD, and Michael Broder, MD

--*Alternative Therapies for Managing Diabetes*, McGraw-Hill, 2000. Revised e-book edition 2011, second print edition 2018.

--*Failure to Atone: Memoirs of a Jungle Surgeon in Vietnam*, 2006, Allen Hassan, MD, JD, DVM, as told to David Drum

--*The Ghosts of War: A Medical Doctor's Guide to Service-Related Disability Letters that Work*, 2010, by Allen Hassan, MD, JD, and David Drum

--*Making the Chemotherapy Decision*, 3rd Edition, Lowell House/Contemporary Books, 2000. 4th Edition e-book 2011, fifth print edition 2018.

--*The Chronic Pain Management Source-book*, Lowell House, 1999. Revised e-book edition 2011, 2014.

Magazine and newspaper articles by David Drum have appeared in *Men's Health, People, USA Today, California Lawyer, Los Angeles Times Magazine,* and *The San Francisco Chronicle.*

The author received an MFA from the University of Iowa, a BA from the University of California at Riverside, and an AA in liberal arts from Brevard College where he served as student body president.

www.daviddrumthewriter.com/

www.burningbookspress.com

INDEX